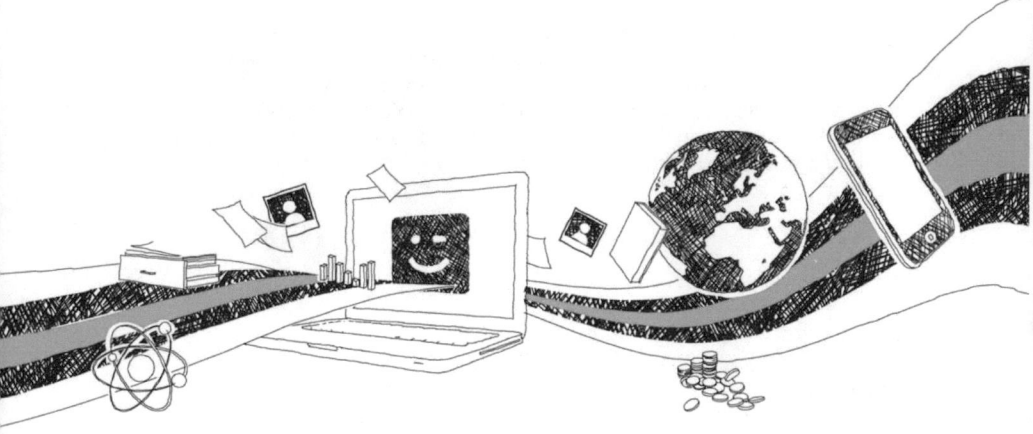
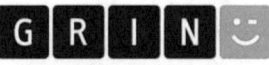

Bibliographic information published by the German National Library:

The German National Library lists this publication in the National Bibliography; detailed bibliographic data are available on the Internet at http://dnb.dnb.de .

Imprint:

Copyright © 2015 GRIN Verlag, Open Publishing GmbH
Print and binding: Books on Demand GmbH, Norderstedt Germany
ISBN: 978-3-668-03624-6

This book at GRIN:

http://www.grin.com/en/e-book/305674/safe-abortion-way-forwards-on-one-of-the-neglected-sexual-and-reproductive

Leonard Kabongo

Safe Abortion. Way forwards on one of the neglected Sexual and Reproductive Health issue

GRIN Publishing

GRIN - Your knowledge has value

Since its foundation in 1998, GRIN has specialized in publishing academic texts by students, college teachers and other academics as e-book and printed book. The website www.grin.com is an ideal platform for presenting term papers, final papers, scientific essays, dissertations and specialist books.

Visit us on the internet:

http://www.grin.com/

http://www.facebook.com/grincom

http://www.twitter.com/grin_com

UNIVERSITY OF MANCHESTER

SCHOOL OF ART, LANGUAGE AND CULTURE

HUMANITARIAN   AND CONFLICT RESPONSE INSTITUTE

POST-GRADUATE CERTIFICATE PROGRAMME IN GLOBAL HEALTH

COURSE TITLE: ETHICS, HUMAN RIGHTS AND HEALTH

MODULE 4 SUMMATIVE ESSAY

Leonard Kabongo

Post-graduate Certificate in Global Health

Table of Contents

1. Introduction

The World Health Organization (1992) defines unsafe abortion as a procedure for terminating a pregnancy that is performed by an individual lacking the necessary skills, or in an environment that does not conform to minimal medical standards, or both. Unsafe abortion is common in places where abortion is illegal. Every year almost 44,000 abortions occur globally and nearly half of them are unsafe whereby almost all unsafe abortions (98 percent) are happening in developing Countries. In Countries where abortion remains unsafe, it is a leading cause of maternal mortality. According to the WHO (2010) unsafe abortions contribute to 13% of all maternal mortality globally and are direct cause of maternal mortality in Sub-Saharan Africa. When comparing women with their counterpart men in Sexual and Reproductive Health, there is no such a high cause of mortality in men. This difference shows the existent gender inequality in most developing Countries. In these settings women are denied access to information, education on safe sex, contraception and are not offered an informed consent on their fertility choices. (Leila, H., 2005). Gender based violence is one of the contributing factor to this inequality that women suffer and this affect their potential development and enjoyment of their right to health including their right to Sexual and Reproductive Health. These universal rights legitimate women to choose whether to conceive or when to form a family. This should have not been difficult to achieve in a World with so much technologies of modern effective contraceptive methods. And the issue of unsafe abortion and its complications could be averted. Conversely this is not the case in the context where legal structures should determine the fate of those who should make decisions for their own lives. The legalization or non-legalization of termination of pregnancy has been a battle ground for Centuries in many Countries across the Globe with different variations in the trends of abortion legal frameworks. In this essay, I will discuss why unsafe abortion is perceived as neglected globally and evaluate the extent to which human rights-based approach can be useful to mitigate this public health problem and conclude with my personal view on this issue.

2. Why and how unsafe abortion is neglected

Unsafe abortions are carried in unsafe conditions where the life of the woman undergoing the procedure is endangered. The magnitude of the issue is not well comprehended due to unreported abortion practices. Global reports estimates are aggregations of Countries reports, research papers and community surveys that are critically analyzed by International Agencies. This limitation shows the level of stigma, sensitivity and socio-cultural aspects attached to the subject. Globally it's estimated that 35 million abortions occur in less developed Countries compare to 7 million in developed Countries annually. (Myers, J.E. and Seif, M.W., 2010).It appears that Countries with high restrictive laws against abortion have more unsafe abortions reported and high complications including high Maternal Mortality Ratio.(Shah, I.H., et al.,2014).Unsafe abortions contribute to 47,000 deaths each year in Sub-Saharan Africa where only two Countries, Cape Verde and South Africa permit abortion on request.

In 1994, the International Conference on Population and Development called for different Governments to engage with women's health by improving accessibility to safe abortion services in places where abortion is legalized and provide post abortion care including management of its complications, counseling, and education on the importance of contraception and information on various contraceptive possibilities. The agreement was imperative for public health and seen as the first step to enhance accessibility of women to Reproductive and Sexual Health Care Services and to enjoy their entitled right to health.

Six years later, WHO strengthened this engagement in the Millennium Development Goals with goal 5 directly targeting women health with clear objectives: firstly to reduce maternal mortality by three quarter between 1990 and 2015, and secondly to achieve universal access to reproductive health services.(United Nations ,2015) .

A decade ago, WHO (2003) published The International Standards and Guidelines for Safe Abortion to mitigate unsafe abortion and its complications in an approach to guide providers in places where safe induced abortion is legally protected.

Further, recently the International Federation of Gynaecologists and Obstetricians (2012) recommended that every woman has the right to a safe medical or surgical induced abortion after an appropriate counseling and that every health care worker has the obligation to provide such services.

Other treaties like the protocol on the right of women in Africa clearly mention the right to abortion and the United Nations special rapporteur on the right to health has pointed out that criminalization of abortion leads to violation of the rights to health. (African Union, 2012). Despite these legal instruments and advocacies, there is wide variation in the trend of abortion laws around the World. Countries may be divided into three categories when considering abortion laws: those with legal permission, Countries with high legal restrictions and Countries with permission on broad medical and social grounds. According to Myers (2010), fifty-six Countries have liberal abortion laws with no reason. Among them 76% are more developed and 31% are less developed. China is included in this group although the law is purely based on procreation control. While these Countries permit abortion without indicating reasons, women still face challenges to access the services. Discrepancies between the *de fore* (laws) and *de facto* (applications of the laws) are not uncommon. In some Countries there is need for several Doctors, parental or spouse consent for a safe abortion. The knowledge and interpretation of the laws by Health Care Workers, the family, and/or the community is another barrier for service accessibility. For example safe abortion is not widely accessible in South Africa, India, Cambodia and Zambia despite liberal legislation. In Countries with high restriction laws women are likely not to receive safe abortion and post abortion care. In these Countries the service is not available or not supported in the public sector. In some instances, the service may be available in the private sector at the woman cost leaving poor women and those that cannot afford with no chance than to opt for unsafe abortion. In Countries with limited legislation, abortion is permitted mostly for reasons like saving the mother or in case of incest or rape.

Globally among 194 Countries, the United Nations (2011) have identified seven reasons of induced abortions among member States: to save the life of the mother (97%), to preserve the mother's physical health (68%), to preserve the mother's mental health

(65%), in case of rape or incest (51%), in case of foetal impairment (51%), for socio-economic reasons (36%) and on request (30%).

For the past decades, significant progress has been seen globally with some Countries adding one reason to another. And the proportion of women of childbearing age leaving in Countries with high restrictive laws have decline from 11% (1999) to 6% (2008). (Myers, J.E. and Seif, M.W., 2010).Nonetheless this reduction is not significant to mitigate the issue of unsafe abortion. Unsafe abortions and its complications still claiming the lives of almost 47,000 women each year in Sub –Saharan Africa where most of Countries have restrictive laws.

Globally unsafe abortion is perceived neglected due to several factors that act in singularity or in symbiosis. The level of advocacy and discussion relating to Women Sexual and Reproductive Health issues at the International and local community tend to be more political or mostly focused on Gender Violence, access to family planning, HIV services including the Protection of Mother to Child Transmission of HIV and campaigns on opposition to forced sterilization. According to Maria de Bruyn (2012), advocacy work to include safe abortion as part of the comprehensive Reproductive and Sexual Health is lagging behind. On my view, Countries' policies relating to abortion are not strengthened enough and voiced out.

Gender, discrimination, stigmatization and victimization of women and human right activists who openly consider abortion as a human right are a reality in most of Countries where abortion laws are restrictive. Women who opt for abortion suffer rejection, abandonment and lack social and family support. Interestingly even in Countries with liberal abortion law, the debate on the topic is always hot and end in perplexity of controversial views among health workers and community. Some Providers consider induced abortion as a major public health problem and that legalization would make a significant advance in women right. They argue better to have an induced abortion legally rather than going for unsafe abortion with all risks attached. Others consider that health care providers should also be given the right to choose whether to work in an abortion clinic or not. (Rehnström L.U. et al, 2015).

In one study in Ghana, human rights arguments were found both going for and against abortion. (Aniteye, P. and Mayhew, S.H., 2013).

Religion and personal beliefs are contributing factors to a lack of decision among Health Care Workers to offer safe abortion services. Some of them fail to make a distinction between their religious beliefs and professional responsibilities. This attitude could be seen as a gap to offer adequate, timely and safe abortion and post abortion care. However, in a study conducted in South Africa Nurses perceived abortion differently depending on whether it's surgical or medical. They think the responsibility of a medical abortion is in the hands of the woman therefore she is answerable to God for her own actions. (Cooper, D.et al, 2005).

In this context, I argue that personal beliefs, values and perceptions should not infringe the safe abortion service whenever indicated or requested especially in an environment of legal protection. Providers with diverse opinions should be able to refer the client to a facility with such a capacity to deliver the service.

The issue of accessibility to the service, the quality of care and training of Health Care Providers in abortion and post abortion care contribute to poor or insufficient service delivery. Adopting abortion liberal law is not enough to mitigate the issue of unsafe abortion. Accessibility of services requires a robust Health Care System with physically accessible clinics, well equipped both with trained human resource and equipments.

Community acceptability can play a major role in abortion care as well. In South Africa, although the abortion Act was promulgated in 1996, Community reactions are mixed despite huge media discussions and talks. There is need for ongoing community education and awareness for improved acceptability. (Harrison, A. et al, 2000)

Rights-based approach can be used to mitigate this complex issue. In the next paragraph I evaluate to what extend this could be made possible.

3. Rights-based approach to mitigate unsafe abortion

Worldwide it is known that 6 in 10 of the 700 million women live in developing Countries (except China and India) where abortion is legally banned or accepted only on basis of saving the mother's life. (Cohen, 2012). Criminalizing abortion does not make it less but unsafe. In Europe, in a Country like Ireland, abortion is illegal but maternal mortality is very low because most of women travel to neighboring Countries to have a safe induced abortion. (United Nations, 2011).Conversely, in Countries like Ethiopia and South Africa, despite the legalization of abortion in 2006 and 1997 respectively, abortion related morbidity and mortality remain high and costly (Cohen, 2012). Women in these Countries have to overcome multiple barriers to have a safe procedure. Ignorance of the law, discrimination, lack of confidentiality and dignified treatment are some of the obstacles to the enjoyment of the right to the attainable higher standard of physical and mental health-the inalienable fundamental human rights. On the other hand, evidence shows that unsafe abortion morbidity and mortality can be lesser with effective contraceptive methods and abolition of coercive and punitive laws against women. In its technical guidance, WHO (2012) further advocates for policy makers to create an enabling environment for women to have access to safe abortion and care and allow them to enjoy the basic fundamental human right .

Abortion still among the leading cause of maternal death along with heaemorhage, sepsis and hypertensive disorders. Reducing maternal mortality is not just an issue of development but also an issue of human rights (Hunt, P. & Brew, J., 2010).Abortion is a critical component of women's sexual and reproductive health and rights. According to Israel (2014) abortion can be important litmus test of whether women's rights are been addressed fundamentally or superficially in a Country. Using the rights-based approach can make a great difference in addressing unsafe abortion. Seven principles form the bedrock of the "human rights-based approach": accountability, participation, transparency, empowerment, sustainability, international cooperation, and non-discrimination.

In 2011, members of Civil Society called for applying human rights-based approach to prevent maternal death and disability. (ICMA, 2014). It was recognized during the meeting that the current practical use of the principles of human-rights based approach is patchy, insufficient and accidental in certain circumstances. It was reiterated that Countries need to double all their efforts to use the human-rights based approach to reduce maternal mortality.

On the other hand, it's important to note that many social determinants of health are rooted in gender inequality that drives unsafe abortion. The risk of gender based violence and the lack of social and legal support, the full dependence on men should be addressed by responsible entities and government bodies for the successful implementation of the rights-based approach to Women's Sexual and Reproductive Health and Rights. Advocacy for women's rights, policy change and abortion laws promulgation in Countries with restrictive legislations, explanation and interpretation of laws at grass root level, integration and empowerment of women in society, a culture of accountability among governments, international cooperation with NGOs, Community based Organizations and Civil Societies, if adopted will be cardinal for the integral management and advancement in the fight against unsafe abortion worldwide.

4. Conclusion

Unsafe abortion is a direct cause of maternal death with 30% of death every year worldwide. Most of the deaths (98%) happen in Developing Countries where abortion laws are restrictive. Evidence show that criminalizing abortion does not reduce its prevalence rather affects its safety. In Sub-Saharan Africa, unsafe abortion claims the lives of 47,000 women each year. Even in Countries in the Region with liberal law like South Africa, Zambia and Ethiopia, safe abortion is not widely accessible. Criminalization, discrimination, stigma, confidentiality, Gender based violence, religious beliefs, cultural beliefs and poor health systems are major contributing factors to negligence of unsafe abortion. Using the rights-based approach by changing policies, human rights advocacy, women empowerment and political will by addressing the social determinants of health focusing on young women and girls can go a long way to make significant progress to address unsafe abortion.

On my view, laws and advocacy alone are limited to address the complex issue of unsafe abortion. There is need for stake holders' engagement. Working along with communities for cultural change, human rights sensitization on Reproductive and Sexual Health Rights for women and discuss laws interpret them as broadly as possible, remove barriers to access for youth, create innovative health systems that are responsive to emerging needs, adopt safe abortion as part of the comprehensive Sexual and Reproductive Health, train Health care workers and strengthen the culture of accountability and confidentiality are critical to mitigate unsafe abortion. In addition, the provision of high-quality post-abortion medical care and post-abortion family planning counseling and contraceptive services are also critical to the prevention of unsafe abortion.

References

1. African Union. (2012). Protocol to the African Charter on Human and Peoples' Rights on the Rights of Women in Africa. http://www.africa-union.org/root/au/ Documents/Treaties/Text/Protocol%20on%20the%20Rights%20of%20Women.p df.

2. Aniteye, P., Mayhew, S.H. (2013). Shaping Legal Abortion Provision in Ghana: Using Policy Theory to Understand Provider-related Obstacles to Policy Implementation. *Health Response and Policy Systems* 11:23.

3. Cohen, S.A. (2012).Access to Safe Abortion in Developing World: Saving Lives While Advancing Rights. *Policy Review.* Volume 15.Number 4.

4. Cooper D, et al. (2005). Medical Abortion: The Possibilities for Introduction in the Public Sector in South Africa. *Reproductive Health Matters;* 13(26*)*:35-43.

5. FIGO. (2012). Ethical Issues in Obstetrics and Gynaecology. October 2012.*FIGO House.* Page 129-130.

6. Harrison, A., Montgomery, E.T., Lurie, M., Wilkinson, D. (2000). Barriers to implementing South Africa's Termination of Pregnancy Act in rural KwaZulu/Natal. *Health Policy Planning. 15(4)*:424-31.

7. International Consortium on Medical abortion, News.2014. http://www.medicalabortionconsortium.org

8. Israel, E. (2014).Advancing Abortion Access in Hostile Environments: A Rights-based Approach. *Pathfinder International.* www.pathfinder.org

9. Leila, H. (2005). Global Progress in Abortion Advocacy and Policy: The Assessment of the Decade since ICPD. *Reproductive Health Matters.* 2005;13:88-100

10. Maria de Bruyn. (2012). HIV, Unwanted Pregnancy and Abortion-Where is the Human Rights Approach. *Reproductive Health Matters.*vol 20,issue 39, page 70-79

11. Myers, J.E. and Seif, M.W. (2010).Global Perspectives of Legal Abortion-Trends Analysis and Accessibility .*Best Practice& Research in Clinical Obstetrics and Gynaecology.* Vol 24,issue 4,page 457-466

12. Paul Hunt and Judith Brew de Mesquita. (2010). Reducing Maternal Mortality: The Contributions of the Right to the Highest Attainable Standard of Health, *UNFPA,* NY. USA.

13. Rehnström, L., U., Gemzell-Danielsson, K., Faxelid, E., & Klingberg-Allvin, M. (2015). Health Care Providers' Perceptions of and Attitudes towards Induced Abortions in Sub-Saharan Africa and Southeast Asia: A Systematic Literature Review of Qualitative and Quantitative Data. *BMC Public Health, 15,* 139. doi:10.1186/s12889-015-1502-2

14. Shah I.H., Ahman, E., Ortayi, N. (2014) .Access to Safe Abortion: Progress and Challenges Since the 1994 International Conference on Population and Development. *Contraception* 90;S39-S48

15. United Nations. (2011). World abortion policies http://www.un.org/esa/population/publications/2011abortion/2011wallchart.pdf

16. United Nations. (2015). http://www.un.org/millenniumgoals/maternal.shtml

17. World Health Organization. (2010).Global Health Report.

18. World Health Organization (2012). Safe Abortion: Technical and Policy Guidance for Health Systems, second ed., Geneva.

19. World Health Organization. (1992).The Prevention and Management of Unsafe Abortion: Report of a Technical Working Group. Geneva. [WHO/MSM/92.5].

YOUR KNOWLEDGE HAS VALUE

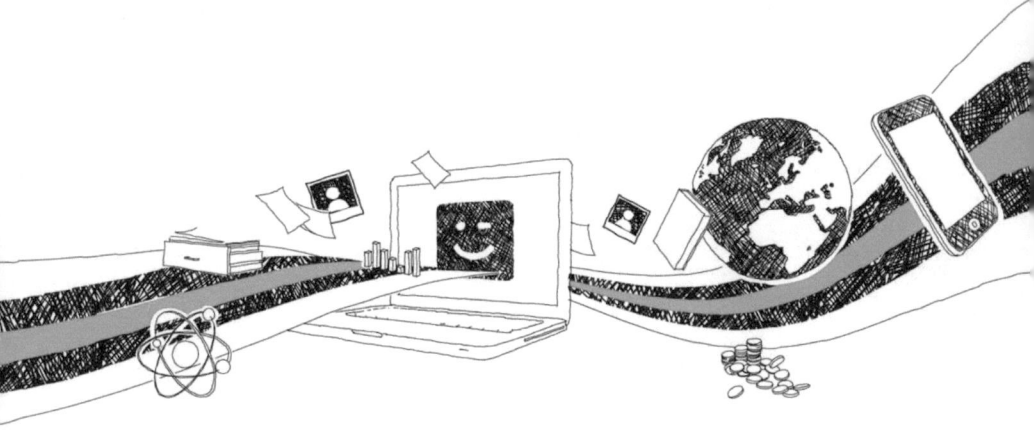

- We will publish your bachelor's and
  master's thesis, essays and papers

- Your own eBook and book -
  sold worldwide in all relevant shops

- Earn money with each sale

Upload your text at www.GRIN.com
and publish for free

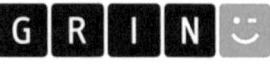